Magic

Stories Behind th

Book 1

Magic Bullets and Beyond

— *Stories Behind the Drugs that Changed the World Series, Book 1*

Guohua An

Fiona-Ann Publishing

Name: Guohua An, author

Title: Magic Bullets and Beyond – Stories Behind the Drugs that Changed the World Series, Book 1 / Guohua An

Identifier: ISBN: 978-1-964623-01-6 (paperback)

My husband Shumin Liu (the editor) and I (the author) dedicate this book to our daughter Fiona Ann Liu.

ABOUT THE AUTHOR

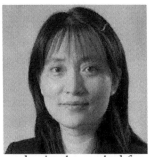

Guohua An, MD, PhD, currently is an Associate Professor in the Department of Pharmaceutical Sciences and Experimental Therapeutics, College of Pharmacy at the University of Iowa. Prior to joining academia, she worked for two and half years at Abbott (currently known as AbbVie), as a Senior Clinical Pharmacokineticist.

Dr. An has been in the pharmaceutical sciences field for 18 years and has published 94 peer-reviewed articles in various top journals in the field. She recently wrote a single author pharmacokinetic textbook, entitled "Essentials in Clinical Pharmacokinetics: Concepts, Dose Optimization, and Biologics", which was released in May 2024 and is available at Amazon.

Dr. An is an editor of Journal of Pharmaceutical Sciences, and she serves as an editorial board member of Journal of Clinical Pharmacology, The AAPS Journal, and Journal of Pharmacokinetics and Pharmacodynamics. In addition to conducting research, she teaches both PharmD students and graduate students.

Besides her beloved pharmaceutical research and teaching, she also loves art and writing.

ii

CONTENTS

PREFACE

I like history, I love stories, and as a pharmaceutical researcher, I have an innate and immense interest in medicines. I never imagined that one day I could link these pieces together and write a book series on the history of drug discovery, a topic full of fascinating stories.

The trigger to write this book was a pharmacokinetics textbook that I wrote earlier this year based on a PharmD course that I have been teaching for years. When I wrote the introduction of biologic products, I did literature search and accidently saw a post talking about the history of smallpox vaccine. It grasped my interest immediately. I dug further and found more and more interesting stories on many other drugs. It's a pity to see many stories, along with the drugs which had (or have) saved millions of lives, gradually faded away as time goes by. In an era of information explosion, these stories are like gems lying on a riverbed. They don't get noticed until you pick them up and look at them closely.

After I enjoyed so much reading those stories and learned a lot from them, I had a strong desire to share them with others. Hence, this book series was born. To prepare this book series, I traced the relevant information from various sources, including drug history books, peer-reviewed journal articles, websites, blogs, DVDs, and magazine interviews. To avoid overwhelming the readers, I intentionally kept each story short and each book thin as the goal was not to write a comprehensive and scholarly book for people in my field. What I really wanted was to write an entertaining and not-boring drug history book series that is suitable for anyone, especially laypersons including teenagers and young adults.

I hope you will like these short stories as much as I do.

Guohua An

June 23, 2024
Iowa City, Iowa

CHAPTER 1

Quinine – From the Sacred Bark
to a Wonder Drug

1.1 The Roman Fever

It was an ancient disease. The earliest records were written more than 3,000 years ago in the *Nei Jing* (the earliest Chinese medical book) and the *Ebers Papyrus* of ancient Egypt, describing the typical symptoms of enlarged spleen, periodic fevers, headache, chills, and fever. The disease had many names, such as intermittent fever, marsh fever, or simply "the fever".

Hippocrates (460-370 BC), a Greek physician, observed that during the harvest time (late summer and autumn) when Sirius, the Dog Star, was dominant in the night sky, fever and misery soon followed. He also noticed that people living near swamps and marshes often suffered from the disease. As the disease was rampant in Rome, the eternal city surrounded by marshland and bogs, it was also called the "Roman fever". It was believed that this fever came from vapors in the swamps during the sickly summer season. Accordingly, Romans called it '*mal'aria*', literally "bad air" in Medieval Italian. Malaria, the name we call the disease today, was unknown in the English language until it was introduced in mid-18th century by an English historian, who during a visit to Rome wrote, "There is a horrid thing called *mal'aria* that comes to Rome every summer and kills one".

For a person who suffers through a cycle of malaria attack, what does it feel like? The most vivid description probably was from Ryszard Kapuscinski, a distinguished journalist and writer, who got malaria and described the disease in his book *The Shadow of the Sun*:

"… If you believe in spirits, you know what it is: someone has pronounced a curse, and an evil spirit has entered you, disabling you and rooting you to the ground. Hence the dullness, the weakness, the heaviness that comes over you. Everything is irritating... ….. It is a sudden, violent onset of cold. A polar, arctic cold. Someone has taken you, naked, toasted in the hellish heat of the Sahel and the Sahara and has thrown you straight into the icy highlands of Greenland or Spitsbergen, amid the snows, winds, and blizzards. …. these tremors and convulsions tossing you around are of a kind that any moment now will tear you to shreds. … He lies in a puddle of sweat, he is still feverish, and he can move neither hand nor foot. Everything hurts; he is dizzy and nauseous. He is exhausted, weak, and limp. Carried by someone else, he gives the impression of having no bones and muscles. And many days must pass before he can get up on his feet again."

Malaria was a terrible disease. Without treatment, it could be deadly. Malaria was not only one of the most ancient diseases but also probably one of the worst that ever hit mankind. It killed people indistinctively: aristocrats, warriors, peasants, cardinals, even Popes.

As Goffredo da Viterbo, a Roman Catholic chronicler, wrote in 1167, "When unable to defend herself by the sword, Rome could defend herself by means of the fever".

For centuries, Europe, Asia, and Africa were ravaged by the terrible marsh fevers, and no one knew exactly what caused the disease, let alone how to treat it. One of the popular medieval treatments involved a sweet apple and an incantation to the three kings who followed the star to Bethlehem: "Cut the apple into three parts. In the first part, write the words Ave Gaspari. In the second write Ave Balthasar, and in the third write Ave Melchior. Then eat each segment early on three consecutive mornings and recite three Our Fathers and three Hail Marys". Another type of medieval cure was passing the disease to animals - for example, a sheep was brought into the bedroom of a fever patient, and holy chants were recited to transfer the illness from the human to the beast. Unfortunately, these popular treatments, without surprise, brought no success.

For a long time, there was no remedy, no cure. At that time, no one knew that, actually, there was a remedy, which our mother nature had placed in a land where had never been reached by malaria, a land waiting for people from the old world to discover. The cure for malaria was hidden in the rainforest's dense jungles of the New World, as the story unfolds in the next section.

1.2 The Miraculous Fever Tree

In the 16th century, as part of the discovery and conquest of the New World, Spanish conquistadors arrived at Inca territory in South America, a place they called Peru, meaning the "land of abundance". There were several legends regarding the discovery of the treatment for malaria.

One legend was about a beautiful Countess of Chinchon, who lay gravely ill with ague in the Viceroy's Palace in Lima, Peru. Deeply worried, her husband, the Count of Chinchon, called the court physician to provide a remedy, but none was at hand. In desperation, the physician obtained a native substance, which was a red powder ground from the bark of a tree growing high in the Andes Mountains. The Countess recovered after taking the remedy, which was called "quina-quina", by the Indian of Peru meaning "bark of barks". When the Countess of Chinchon returned to her homeland Spain, she brought the red power with her, which came to be known in Europe as the "Countess' powder".

Many years later, a Swedish naturalist named the tree from which the bark was obtained *Cinchona* in her honor. Despite the spelling error (the first *h* from the name was left off), Cinchona remains enshrined as the name for the fever bark tree. The story of Countess of Chinchon was circulated for 300 years till the diary of the Count and viceroy was discovered in the early 20th century, which revealed that his wife never had malaria and had been in good health her entire time in Peru.

There is another legend, which goes with a fatally ill man with high fever. He was lost in the jungle. He drank water from a shallow pool and then fell asleep. When he woke up, he was cured. All he remembered was that the water he drank was awfully bitter and there were fallen cinchona trees lying in it. Although it was unclear if this legend remains true, the common part of the above two stories is that there was a miraculous fever tree that saved people's lives.

The Peruvian trees, which has been called quina-quina, or most commonly today, Cinchona, grow in a narrow swath on the slopes and valleys of the Andes – they do not grow lower than 2,500 ft or higher than 9,000 ft above the sea level. The benefit of the bark of the Cinchona tree had long been recognized by indigenous peoples before the arrival of the Spanish. The original inhabitants drank a broth made from cinchona bark when they had shivers from the cold. When the Spanish Jesuits saw the natives using a particular bark to stop shivers, they made the connection: maybe the same ingredient of the bark could be used for the shivers caused by malaria, and they were right.

Spanish Jesuits brought the dried bark back to Rome in early 17th century, which is why it is also called "Jesuits powder" or "Jesuits bark". The first written record in Europe about a "miraculous" malaria remedy discovered in the jungles of the New World appeared in 1630s, and samples of the Jesuits powder appeared in Europe around the same time. By the 1640s, Jesuits

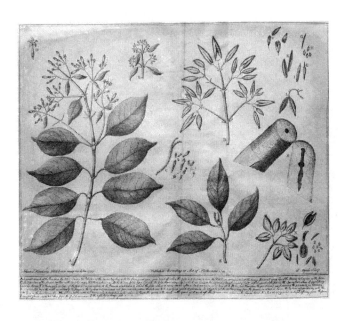

Peruvian tree, which has been called quina-quina, cascarilla, or most commonly today, Cinchona.

had established trade routes to deliver cinchona bark throughout Europe.

Cinchona bark was truly a game changing treatment. Based on the record, six cardinals died of malaria during the papal conclave in 1620s. Thirty years later, not one cardinal died during the papal conclave. Because of the miraculous bark powder, 1655 was the

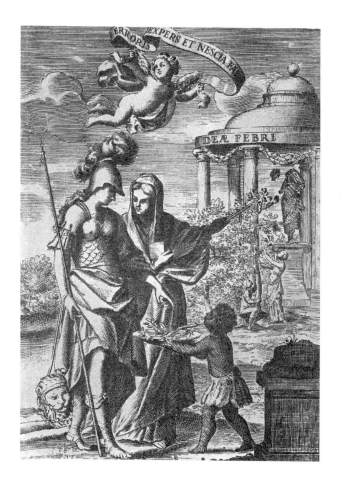

Peru offers a branch of cinchona to Science (17th century engraving). Cinchona genus is the source of Peruvian bark, an important historical remedy against malaria.

first year when not one citizen of Rome died of malaria. As an Italian physician stated in 1650, "This bark has proven more precious to mankind than all the gold and silver the Spaniards obtained from South America".

After reading here, you might think that, from the 1650s onward, no country in Europe would suffer from malaria since the trade routes of cinchona bark had been well established. Then you would be wrong. A few countries, including England, were against cinchona bark for many years, and they paid a deep price, at the cost of both lives and gold, prior to their final acceptance of Jesuits' Bark; this interesting story is told in the next section.

1.3 The Successful Charlatan and His Secret Recipe

When this miraculous Jesuit's powder came to Europe, not everyone was happy with it. For Protestants, it was hard for them to accept that the cure for the most ancient and deadly disease came from Jesuits, their religious rivals. All Protestants immediately rejected the powder, and they called it

"Jesuit plot". In addition, the bark was awfully bitter. "We knew it, those Jesuits are trying to poison us!". In countries dominated by Protestants, such as England, Holland, and Germany, pretty much everybody refused to use it. As a result, even many years after the cinchona bark entered Europe, the death rate of malaria did not drop in these countries; many people died due to untreated malaria.

Another layer of resistance came from the medicine field due to the concerns of unknown principle of action, unclear dosage and treatment duration. The environment of medicinal uncertainty, together with the religious resistance, bred many charlatans and hucksters, among whom the most famous one was an English apothecary named Robert Talbor.

Robert Talbor, born in 1642, was just a quack, and he had no proper medical training. He went to Essex in 1668 and developed his secret recipe for malaria, a recipe he named "Pyretologia". In 1672, he wrote a slim publication, entitled "Pyretologia: A Rational Account of the Cause and Cure of Agues", which was more like a marketing brochure promoting his miracle drug than a scientific paper. In this article, he described how to administer Pyretologia in detail, but only vaguely mentioned that the drug was a preparation of four vegetables, whereof two were foreign and the other domestic. He specifically warned against the use of chinchona bark:

"… let me advise the world beware of all palliative cures and especially that known the name of Jesuits' Powder, as it is given by unskillful hands for I have seen dangerous effects follow the taking of the medicine uncorrected and unprepared."

When physicians requested him to provide more complete information of his mystery Pyretologia, Talbor responded that he deserved to be compensated before releasing the ingredients of the drug:

"I intend hereafter to publish a larger, and fuller account of my particular method, and medicine, not being willing to conceal such useful remedies from the world any longer, than till I have made some little advantage myself, repay that charge and trouble I have at in the search and study of so great and unheard of secrets."

When he was asked the cause of malaria fever, his response was:

"Gentleman, I do not pretend to know anything about fever except that it is a disease which all you others do not know how to cure, but which I cure without fail."

The mystery Pyretologia turned Talbor from a poor man into a famous, successful, and rich one. Using his secret recipe, Talbor successfully cured many aristocrats and royalty, including King Charles II of England and the son of King Louis XIV of France. It was an incredible journey. He was appointed as a physician of two kings and became a celebrated healer of the royal courts in London, Madrid, and Paris. King Louis XIV was thrilled with the miracle cure and offered to buy the ingredients with 2,000 gold livre (French pounds) and a lifetime pension, a reward that was hard to turn down. Talbor accepted the offer with one condition: the ingredients of his wonderful secret recipe would only be made public after his death. The King agreed, and it did not take long to wait - Talbor died 2 years later, in 1681. Apparently, Talbor did not get a chance to enjoy his royal reward very long. One

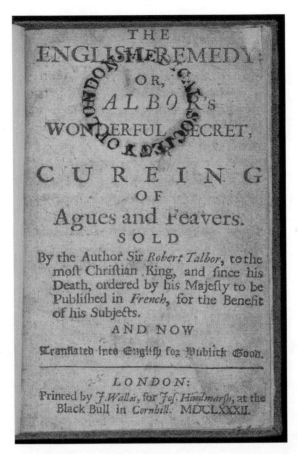

The English Remedy: Talbor's Wonderful Secret for Curing of Agues and Feavers (1682). Robert Talbor sold the secrets of his malaria treatment to King Louis XIV for 2,000 guineas, on condition that they would not be published until after his death. In 1682, Talbor's remedy was published in French; the English translation appeared in the same year.

year after his death, the key component of Pyretologia was identified and released (as shown in the figure on page 14). Guess what was the secret ingredient? Jesuits' Powder – the ground bark of the cinchona tree.

1.4 Quinine and the Yellow Cinchona

The active ingredient in Talbor's secret recipe was certainly an easy one to figure out. In contrast, identifying the active component of the cinchona bark was a much more challenging task. It remained unknown until Pierre Pelletier and Joseph Caventou, two accomplished French pharmacists and scientists, isolated it in 1820, almost 200 years after Jesuits powder was first introduced in Europe in the 1630s.

This important work was done in their laboratory in the back of a Parisian apothecary shop. There are several different kinds of cinchona bark. Pelletier and Caventou studied extracts from six varieties of the cinchona tree, including the grey cinchona, yellow cinchona, and red cinchona. The substance that made them famous was found in the bark of the yellow cinchona. The isolation process was not easy. The bark

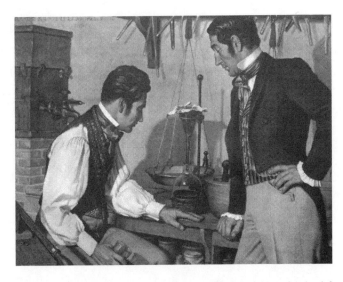

Pierre Pelletier and Joseph Caventou isolated quinine from bark of the Cinchona Tree in back of their pharmacy (about 1820).

powder was first mixed with alcohol, then rinsed with a hot solution of hydrochloric acid, leading to a purified extract which was a white powder after being washed and dried. Later steps involved dissolving the white powder in alcohol. After the clear alcohol extract was evaporated, the undissolved part was a pale-yellow gummy substance, a bitter-tasting alkaloid. They named it quinine based on the Indian word "quina-quina", the native name of the cinchona tree.

Interestingly, when they used the same procedure for grey cinchona, the substance they obtained would not be quinine but another alkaloid, cinchonine. On the other hand, both quinine and cinchonine are present in the red cinchona tree.

Considering the enormous population infected with malaria in the 19th century, Pelletier and Caventou could have been very rich had they patented their method of quinine isolation. However, they gave up a fortune in doing so and chose a different route – instead of filing a patent, they invited other researchers to verify the therapeutic properties of quinine as soon as possible. For such an important discovery, the only money they had ever received was a small sum of 10,000 francs from the French Institute of Science in 1827.

Pelletier and Caventou's quinine extraction method became well-known and was soon used by many pharmacists. Based on their method, many firms began to manufacture quinine commercially. The demand for cinchona bark skyrocketed. By the 1840s, millions of tons of cinchona bark were exported to Europe from the Andean republics. The native suppliers chopped

down one tree after another. Because of reckless
stripping of the forests, cinchona trees became
increasingly scarce. It became more difficult to find
species with sufficient quinine content in the bark.

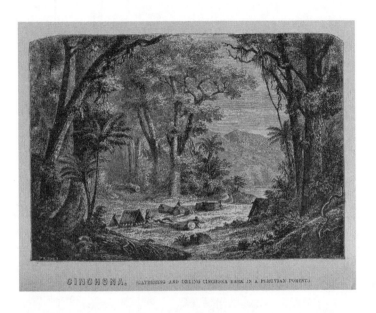

*The gathering and drying of cinchona bark in a Peruvian forest.
As Europeans hired locals to harvest more quinine to fuel their
colonial pursuits, cinchona trees became increasingly scarce.*

In 1844, Bolivia passed laws to prohibit the collection and export of seeds and plants without a license; the aim was to protect their monopoly and prevent smuggling because 15% of the country's tax revenue came from bark exports. The two main colonial powers, England and Holland, were unhappy with the situation and wanted to move the cultivation of cinchona trees to their colonial territories. During their race to see who would be the first to establish cinchona plantations outside of South America, stories came along, as shown in the next section.

1.5 The Unlucky Adventurer and His Faithful Servant

The English decided to cultivate cinchona trees in India, while the Dutch chose Java, Indonesia. Now all they needed was cinchona seeds. This task, seemed simple at first glance, turned out to be not easy at all. First, there are many different species of Cinchona trees, and not all have high yield of quinine. Second, Cinchona trees grew in inaccessible tropical forests on the slopes of the Andes mountains. The variable climate was often accompanied with thick mist, sunshine alternating with showers and storms, and near freezing temperatures. Consequently, seed collection was relied on the Indians, called cascades.

While eventually both the English and the Dutch managed to procure cinchona seeds and planted them in their respective colonial territories, unfortunately, the Cinchona trees they planted had low quinine yield. For example, the trees planted in British India had a quinine content of only 2% in their bark. In the end, a million Cinchona trees were destroyed because the entire British venture was found to be unprofitable. The situation of Dutch was no better. Therefore, in the first round, both the English and the Dutch ended in failure.

Now enters the main character of our story, Charles Ledger (1818-1905), an unlucky adventurer and a legendary figure. In his early career, Ledger worked as a trader in alpaca wools in Peru. In 1853, a group of Australian clients were interested in bringing a herd of alpacas from Peru to Australia to raise and breed in the new homeland. At that time, the export of alpacas from Peru to Europe was strictly prohibited, and anyone violating it could end in prison. The clients approached

Ledger and promised him generous remuneration, including around 9,800 acres of land to set up a farm in Australia. Ledger was resourceful, tenacious, and knew how to bypass the prohibition. He decided to take the risk. Ledger signed the contract, bought the animals, hired herdsmen, and embarked on a 6,800-mile journey across the South America, a journey took him nearly six years. Despite numerous challenges and tough situations, he successfully carried 256 alpacas to Australia.

However, during these six years, many things had happened in Australia. The original clients either had financial disaster or left Australia. Suddenly, nobody was interested in breeding alpacas. Ledger did not receive the land promised to him, and no one wanted the alpacas when he tried to sell them in an auction. In the end, he had to give up. He wrote, "On the faith of promises made in this country, I undertook every risk – did succeed – and am ruined!".

Ledger returned to Peru in 1860. He quit the alpaca business and chose a completely different commodity this time. As he was living in the cinchona area for a long time, he was able to differentiate between the less and more active barks. Realizing the global high demand for Jesuits' bark, he sent his servant Manuel Incra Mamani, a Bolivian cascarillero, to search for cinchona seeds. From upland of Bolivia, Mamani knew 29 varieties of Cinchona by the shape and size of the leaves, and by the color of the flowers and bark. The target was a stand of 50 huge Cinchona trees that Ledger and Mamani had seen in flower in Bolivia 9 years earlier (1851) during the exploration of a mountainous passage for alpacas. It took Mamani 5 years to collect the seeds because the first 4 years frosts destroyed the flowers and prevented the ripening of the fruits to produce seeds. Finally in 1865, he succeeded, and walked more than 1000 miles from Bolivia to bring the seeds to Ledger.

These were high quality seeds. Ledger carefully dried the seeds, hid them among some chinchilla pelts, and sent them to his brother, who lived in London. His brother attempted to sell them to the British government, but the government was not interested. He approached several other potential customers and got rejections one after another. Eventually, the Dutch consulate general in London bought some with 100 Dutch guldens (about £20). The seeds took root in Java, and the cinchona trees had a much higher quinine content than any species before it. The disinterest of the English gave the Dutch a monopoly on quinine trade. Purchasing Ledger and Mamani's cinchona seeds with 100 guldens has been considered one of the best trades in history. The Dutch earned unprecedented profits for several decades. It was considered the most effective crop monopoly of any kind in all history.

The end of the story was rather miserable and depressing. Shortly after Mamani delivered the seeds to Ledger, he was seized by the Bolivia officials. For refusing to tell whom he had been working for, Mamani was imprisoned, beaten, and starved. He died shortly after he was set free. Ledger was grief-stricken by Mamani's death. He stopped the seed collection and cared for Manuel's family with money and other help. Ledger eventually retired in Australia where he received a miserable pension from the Dutch. He died in 1905 in poverty, and his death passing largely unnoticed.

Later, this high-yielding species was named *Cinchona Ledgeriana* in his honor. In 1994, a tombstone was erected in his memory and the inscription says "Here lies Charles Ledger. He gave quinine to the world".

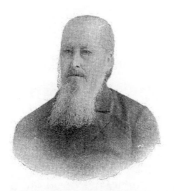

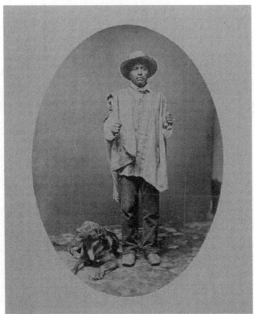

Charles Ledger (upper photo) and Manuel Incra Mamani (lower photo)

There is, however, no monument to Manuel Incra Mamani, Ledger's faithful servant, who spent five hard years gathering high quality seeds in the harsh rainforests and paid the price of his life.

1.6 The Mosquitoes with Spotted Wings

For a long time, the cause of the malaria was thought to be the poisonous vapors ("bad air") from swamps. With the advances in bacteriology in the second half of the 19th century, the bad air theory was replaced with a new thought – the disease was due to the bacteria near stagnant and dirty water entering the human body via inhalation. This bacteria theory, seemed convincing, was challenged by Alphonse Laveran, a French Army physician. In 1880, when he examined a drop of fresh blood from a soldier infected with malaria, he saw several transparent mobile filaments emerging from a spherical body. He realized that he was looking at alive animals instead of bacteria. He did further investigations and named the one-celled beast *Oscillaria malariae*. As the discovery was so unusual, at that time no one believed him. The scientific community unanimously rejected it.

As always, truth prevails. It is just a matter of time. Several years later, Laveran's discovery of the parasite was confirmed by other researchers. While it was clear that malaria was caused by parasites, instead of bacteria or bad air, the part that remained unknown was the transmission of the parasite. The missing piece was filled by Ronald Ross, a military doctor from India, with the help from his teacher and mentor Patrick Manson in London.

Manson suspected that mosquitoes were the culprit of malaria. To prove Manson's theory, Ross caught mosquitos, let them bite malaria patients, then killed and observed mosquitos under a microscope. Most experiments failed at the beginning; Ross saw nothing abnormal. At that time, neither Ross nor Manson knew that, among various kinds of mosquitoes in the *Anopheles* genus, only a small percentage of them could transmit malaria parasite from human to human.

The lucky date arrived on August 19, 1897. His assistant brought Ross a few mosquitos with spotted wings. As usual, Ross convinced one of his malaria patients to let the mosquitos bite him. When he dissected and observed the mosquitos under the microscope, he saw a malarial parasite (plasmodia) inside the stomach of a mosquito. He was thrilled and wrote the following poem the next day after this important discovery:

This Day relenting God
Hath placed withing my hand
A wondrous thing; and God
Be praised. At his command,

Seeking his secret deeds
With tears and toiling breath,
I find thy cunning seeds,
O million-murdering Death

I know this little thing
A myriad men will save.
O Death, where is thy sting?
Thy victory, O Grave?

The mosquito with the spotted wings, the culprit of malaria transmission, belongs to a specific species in the *Anopheles* genus, known as *Anopheles gambiae.* Later, Ross also found plasmodia in the salivary gland of the mosquito. With these findings, he was able to put all pieces together: The mosquito sucked the blood of a sick man, plasmodia were transferred to its stomach. The same mosquito stung the second person. Consequently, the plasmodia were transferred from the saliva of the mosquito to this person who had been healthy. The blood of the second person, who became sick, served as a new source to feed more mosquitos and spread the disease. Later, a zoology professor, Giovanni Batista Grassi, confirmed Ross's findings with elegant human clinical studies. In addition, Grassi discovered that only female mosquitos with spotted wings could transmit the disease.

Once the parasite entered humans, it first migrated to the liver, where it underwent a multiplication in hepatocytes. The numerous parasites generated led to the rupture of their host cells. As a result, they escaped into the blood, where they entered red blood cells for further multiplication. Eventually, the rapid

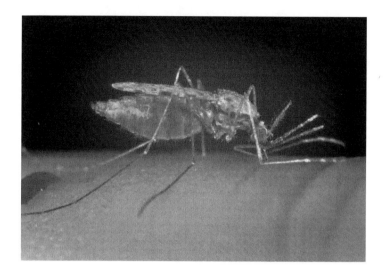

This image depicts a female Anopheles gambiae mosquito, which was in the process of obtaining a blood meal through the skin of its human host. A. gambiae is a known malaria vector.

multiplication resulted in the rupture of the red blood cells. Each burst was associated with a cycle of fever, and the fever spike may reach up to 41°C. Several such amplification cycles could occur, with each being characterized by a wave of fever.

As commented by Henry Havelock Ellis, an English-French physician, writer, and social reformer, in 1920, "If you would see all of Nature gathered up at one point, in all her loveliness, and her skill, and her deadliness, and her sex, where would you find a more exquisite symbol than the Mosquito?".

1.7 Gin and Tonic

Quinine had a transformative impact on human civilization as it made malaria-ridden lands inhabitable. Without it, Western colonization would fail due to the huge swaths of South America, North America, Africa, and the Indian subcontinent. Quinine was packed into the bags of everyone (soldiers, government officials, merchants, etc.) involved in the settling in Africa, a place used to be known as "white man's grave".

In December 1941, the Japanese attacked Pearl Harbor, which triggered World War II. Next year, the Japanese invaded Java, where 90% of the world's supply of quinine came from. This led to the global shortage of quinine. Consequently, there was a big push by the U.S. military to synthesize quinine and develop new antimalarial drugs.

Today, quinine has been replaced by new antimalarial drugs and is no longer a first-line drug. It is used occasionally in the treatment of severe falciparum malaria. Interestingly, quinine holds a spot in the food industry - it is used in a low amount as the bitter element in soft drinks such as tonic water. An eight-ounce glass of tonic water contains roughly 20 mg quinine, which is about one-tenth of the amount in one quinine tablet. Among different brands of tonic water, one was named after Charles Ledger (the unlucky adventurer mentioned in section 1.5) – *Ledger's Tonic.*

You may have heard of a classic cocktail named "gin and tonic". Its history can be traced back to early 19th century when British soldiers stationed in India and were prescribed to take doses of the prophylactic quinine in order to fight malaria. Since quinine is very bitter, it was then mixed with sugar, citrus extracts and carbonated water; this was the birth of Indian Tonic. Later, to further make the medicine more palatable, gin was mixed with the tonic water to improve the taste and meanwhile mask the bitter flavor of quinine. As time went by, gin and tonic gained popularity and became a classic cocktail enjoyed worldwide.

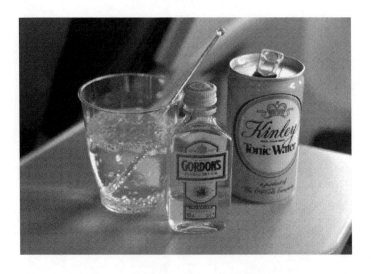

Gin & tonic (containing, of course, quinine)

The history of quinine is a saga containing many elements: exploration, bravery, generosity, greed, misfortune, adventure, and the colonial ambitions of the European powers. From the sacred bark to a wonder drug, quinine changed human history. When we sip our gin and tonic, we should raise a glass and give thanks to all who had played important roles in the quest for quinine: the Jesuits, Pelletier & Caventou, Ledger & Mamani, and many others...

CHAPTER 2

Salvarsan - The Magic Bullet

2.1 One Step from Hell

In August 1494, King Charles VIII of France launched an invasion of Italy with an army of 50,000 soldiers, mostly mercenaries – Gascon, Swiss, Italian, Flemish, and Spanish. The army was accompanied by 800 camp followers, including cooks and prostitutes. It seemed to be an easy-to-win battle at the beginning. Charles' army crushed all resistance from intervening

Italian cities and in February 1495 took Naples, where the French soldiers indulged in a long run of celebration and debauchery.

The invading troops soon fell ill. The disease started with angry red ulcers on the genitals, followed by fresh-pink rash on the body, then progressed to a fever, with joint and muscle pains. The victims often had pustules covering the body from the head to the knees, causing flesh to fall from their faces, making them look like demons from hell. As described by Joseph Grunbeck, a German historiographer, in the end of 15th century, the disease was "so cruel, so distressing, so appalling that until now nothing so horrifying, nothing more terrible or disgusting, has ever been known on this earth."

This terrible disease was new. No one had seen it before. The French troops called it "the disease of Naples" or "the Italian disease", while Italians called it "the French disease", blaming each other for it. This disease forced the withdrawal of Charles' army because many soldiers were too sick to fight. During their retreat from Italy, the undisciplined troops, consisting of mercenaries from many parts of Europe, carried the disease back to their respective homelands. As a result, the disease spread rapidly through Europe. Within 10 years, the disease was epidemic- it was carried to Hungary, Russia, Africa, Middle East, India, and later China. Eventually, the disease reached every continent.

Along with its widespread coverage, the disease earned several new names; usually people named it after an enemy or a country they thought responsible for it. For example, the Russian called it "the Polish disease"; the Polish and the Persians called it the 'Turkish disease'; the Turkish called it the "Christian disease', and so on.

In 1530, Girolamo Fracastoro, a poet, mathematician and physician, wrote an epic Latin poem 'Syphilis, or the French disease', which described a mythical shepherd named Syphilus who kept the flocks of King Alcithous. One year, a drought affected Syphilus' people. Syphilus insulted the Sun-God by blaspheming against him and blaming the god for the drought. The Sun-God was angry and punished Syphilus and his people by striking them down with a disgusting and odorous new disease. This poem was the origin of the term "syphilis", which is the name of the disease we call today.

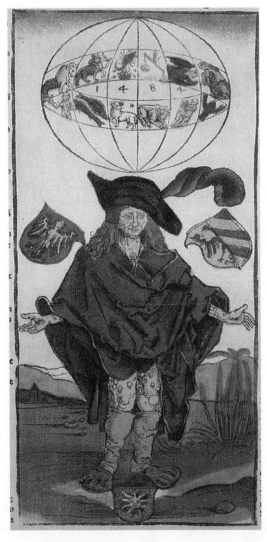

Wood cut of a Syphilitic Man, Albrecht Dürer, 1496

2.2 As the Story Goes

The mysterious epidemic struck terror into all hearts by the rapidity of its spread and the ravages it made. Where did syphilis come from? Surprisingly, till now, more than 500 years after the Naples outbreak, its precise origin is still being debated. One prominent theory is that it was from the New World, and it was brought to the old world by Christopher Columbus and his sailors after they visited the Americas. The crew, upon arrival in Spain in 1493, disbanded and some of them joined the army of Charles VIII.

Fifty to a hundred years after its appearance in Naples, the severity and fatality of syphilis were reduced. Different from the acute and explosive symptoms seen in the early 1500s, the disease was more chronic, with several distinct phases. The first phase, also known as the chancre stage, included pea-sized ulcers, or "pocks" occurring on the lips, fingers, and/or genitals. The chancre usually disappeared within several weeks, leaving a small and inconspicuous scar.

The second phase, also known as disseminated stage, usually developed several weeks, and in some cases more than a year, after the chancre. The typical symptoms included headache, sore throat, fever, rash all over the body, and night bone pains. The highly infectious second phase usually did not last long, giving patients a false impression that they fully recovered.

After a long latent period, lasting months and even years, the last phase (tertiary stage) came, which was a nightmare - the victims got destructive ulcers appearing in the skin, muscles, lungs, and eyes, causing disfigurement; the spinal cord and brain were affected, leading to paralysis, epileptic seizures, and insanity.

Many historical figures had syphilis, including rulers, political figures, musicians, and artists, etc. One example is Ivan IV Vasilyevich (1530-1584), an infamous tsar of Russia, who was commonly known as "Ivan the Terrible" in history. The Soviet Union exhumed his tomb and found typical lesions in his bones, indicating that he was a victim of tertiary syphilis. Ivan ruled Russia wisely and humanely in the early years. In the later years, he slaughtered thousands of people. One of the victims was his own son and heir, whom he killed using a steel-pointed staff. The madness, insanity, and paranoia of Ivan the Terrible were believed to be the consequences of his neurosyphilis.

Since its first outbreak in 1495, syphilis remained to be one of the most feared diseases in Europe for several centuries. Many people considered it a divine punishment for sin. Syphilis resulted in mass closure of public bathhouses in the 1500s because the new disease scared away clients. By the end of the 19th century, 10% of the population of Europe was estimated to be infected with syphilis. In addition, one third of all patients in mental hospitals could trace their neurological symptoms to tertiary syphilis.

2.3 Holy Wood and Mercury

In the 16th century, guaiacum (holy wood) was a popular treatment for syphilis because it came from Hispaniola, an island in the Caribbean, where Columbus had landed in the New World; this made people believed that God had provided a cure in the same location where the disease originated. The use of holy wood was described in Fracastoro's 1530 poem:

"…drink the first potion by the beaker twice a day: in the morning at sunrise and by the light of the evening star. The treatment lasts until the moon completes its orbit and after the space of a month

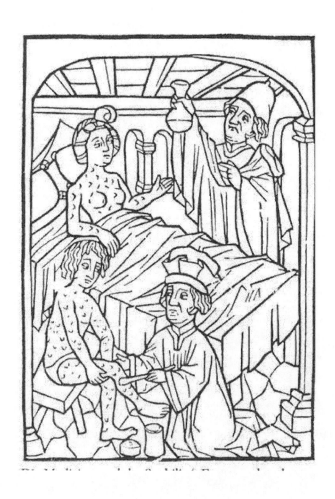

An early medical illustration of people with syphilis, Vienna, 1498.

conjoins again with the sun. The patient must remain in a room protected from wind and cold, so that frost and smoke do not diminish the effect of the remedy." Unfortunately, the holy wood from the New World, an exotic remedy, was not effective as a cure for syphilis.

Another common and long-standing treatment for syphilis was mercury. Usually, patients were scheduled in a hot, stuffy room, and rubbed vigorously with the mercury ointment several times a day. While mercury had some ameliorative effect and thus was better than the useless holy wood, it was quite toxic, and many patients died of mercurial poisoning rather than the disease itself. Nevertheless, since mercury was the only meaningful option, the treatment would go on for years, which gave rise to the saying, "A night with Venus, and a lifetime with mercury".

For a long time, there was no effective treatment for syphilis. This situation was about to change when a seemingly unrelated event occurred in the late 19 century – the rapid rising of synthetic dye industry in Europe, as the story mentioned in the next section.

2.4 The Wonder of Aniline Dyes

Before the mid-19th century, fabrics were stained using natural dyes made from plants and animals. The vibrant colors, such as Tyrian purple made from predatory sea snails, were very costly and incredibly difficult to produce; fabrics stained with these colors were mainly reserved for aristocrats and royalty.

For average people, dressed like royalty would sound like a daydream. In 1856, an English teenager named William Henry Perkin (1838-1907) turned the dream into reality. It started with a serendipitous discovery. One day Perkin performed a chemistry experiment in his apartment to try to synthesize quinine using coal tar products, an activity similar to a high school student playing with a home chemistry kit nowadays. The experiment failed as Perkin got a black solid substance at the bottom of his beaker instead of the expected white quinine crystals. Luckily, before he tossed it away, he first dissolved it in alcohol. A solution with beautiful lustrous purplish color was generated, which later was called 'aniline violet', 'Perkin's purple' or 'mauveine'. This was the world's first synthetic dye.

The accidental discovery of beautiful mauveine was probably one of the most successful mistakes in history. Perkin, who had an interest in painting and photography, immediately realized the potential of this purple dye. He did further tests and found that it dyed silk in a way which was stable when washed or exposed to light. The result was so promising that Perkin filed a patent when he was still only 18 years old. He quit college, set up a dye factory, and soon became rich.

After the discovery of mauveine, many new aniline dyes were discovered later by dye companies, including a variety of shades of purples and magentas, yellows, blues, and pinks. These colors, much more vibrant and intense than any available from the traditional natural dyes, became very fashionable. Even better, the major source of the raw material, coal tar, was an abundant by-product of the process for making coal gas and coke, which means that synthetic aniline dyes would cost significantly less than the traditional expensive natural dyes.

Perkin's discovery revolutionized the dye industry from the late 1850s onwards. The fabrics with aniline dyes were characterized by an unprecedented brilliance and intensity which delighted all customers. For the

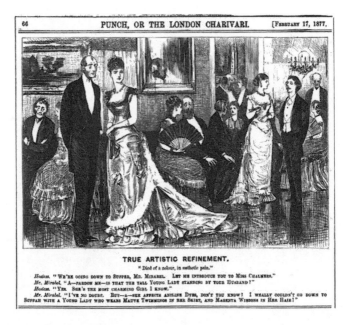

TRUE ARTISTIC REFINEMENT.

"Died of a colour, in æsthetic pain."

Hostess. "We're going down to Supper, Mr. Mirabel. Let me introduce you to Miss Chalmers."
Mr. Mirabel. "A—pardon me—is that the tall Young Lady standing by your Husband?"
Hostess. "Yes. She's the most charming Girl I know."
Mr. Mirabel. "I've no doubt. But—a—she affects aniline Dyes, don't you know! I really couldn't go down to Supper with a Young Lady who wears Mauve Trimmings in her Skirt, and Magenta Ribbons in her Hair!"

The craze for aniline dyes, described in this cartoon published in the satirical journal 'Punch' in 1877. Bright colors had firmly infiltrated 'respectable' fashion.

first time, even people with low income could afford clothes with rich hues. Everyone could dress like royalty. The craze for aniline dyes was described in the weekly journal *All The Year Round* in 1859, 'As I look out of my window now, the apotheosis of Perkin's purple seems at hand - purple hands wave from open carriages; purple hands shake each other at street doors; purple hands threaten each other from opposite sides of the street'. It appeared that all social classes were sporting this vivid shade. Bright garments flooded the streets....

The discovery of synthetic dyes and the public's thirst for color led to the rapid rising of the synthetic dye Empire. In addition to the high-tech products for their core market, over the years dye companies generated many spinoff products/applications, such as the use of off-the-shelf dyes in staining cells, etc. A German scientist was fascinated with synthetic dyes, and with years effort he developed a miracle drug (with a dye component) for syphilis in 1910. His name is Paul Ehrlich. The first outbreak of syphilis was in 1495. Four hundred and fifteen years later, finally a drug that can cure syphilis was born. It was indeed a history-altering discovery. The story of Dr. Paul Ehrlich and his miracle drug is provided in the next section.

2.5 A Scientific Genius and His Magic Bullet

Paul Ehrlich was born on March 14th, 1854 to a middle-class Jewish family. When he was in medical school, he was never viewed as an outstanding student because his professors believed that he put too much time on tissue staining, a pointless distraction in their opinion. When one of his professors introduced Ehrlich to guest speaker Robert Koch, an eminent physician, he said, "That is little Ehrlich. He is very good at staining, but he will never pass his examinations".

It did not take long to prove that his professors were wrong. Through tissue-staining investigations, Ehrlich, who was just a graduate student back then, discovered a new cell type, which he named master cells. The new staining and diagnostic methods he developed, using the recently discovered aniline-derived dyes, laid a foundation for modern hematology. He obtained a doctorate with a dissertation in 1878, entitled "Contributions to the Theory and Practice of Histological Staining".

Over the years, Ehrlich noticed that the uptake of different dyes varied in different tissues, which made him come up with a provocative idea: what if there is a double-duty dye, which can stain a certain type of pathogen but not the host, and meanwhile was toxic to that pathogen? Ehrlich called it *Zauberkugel* -"magic bullet". With that concept in mind, he started to search for such magic bullets.

The first pathogen he targeted was the parasite that causes malaria. With extensive screening, he found that methylene blue, which showed some toxicity to the malaria pathogen, only stained the parasite but not human tissue. However, although he was able to cure two malaria patients with some success, this therapy was not superior to quinine, then in wide use. His team then investigated numerous synthetic dyes on various other pathogens. To his great disappointment, the substantial efforts yielded little progress.

After multiple rounds of failure, Ehrlich realized that it was too difficult to find a dye to fulfill the double duty task. So, he modified his theory. In his revised vision, the magic bullet would contain the following two partners linked together via chemical synthesis: a toxin, which has the capability to kill a pathogen, and a dye, which only stains the pathogen but not the host. In this case, even if the toxin was harmful to humans,

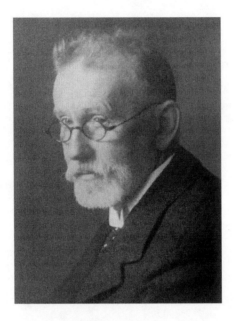

Paul Ehrlich (1854 -1915)

it won't cause toxicity as the dye attached to it acted as a navigator or guide.

With this updated concept, Ehrlich used arsenic as the toxin and conjugated it with a dye, creating a new compound called atoxyl. Initially he attempted to use it to treat Chagas disease, which was caused by a parasite known as *Trypanosoma cruzi*. His team created and tested hundreds of variants of atoxyl, and all compounds failed - they were either ineffective, or effective but very toxic to the host.

Facing a dead end, Ehrlich decided to switch to another disease. In the meantime, *Treponema pallidum*, the pathogen that causes syphilis, was identified in 1905 by a zoologist and a dermatologist. Without a second thought, Ehrlich tested his conjugated compounds to syphilis. His team prepared hundreds of compounds, each with a unique number, and tested them in hundreds of animals. The first 605 compounds failed. The next compound, which was labeled "606", was found to be both effective and safe. Further clinical studies also confirmed the animal results. Ehrlich named it "salvarsan" - the first man-made antibiotic, the first magic bullet Ehrlich so earnestly sought, was born in 1909.

Salvarsan was manufactured by Hoechst AG, a German company that provided Ehrlich many dyes over the years, and marketed to the public in 1910. Physicians and desperate patients besieged the Hoechst manufacture site for the lifesaving "magic bullet". Almost overnight, Ehrlich became a world celebrity. When he was congratulated on the success of Salvarsan,

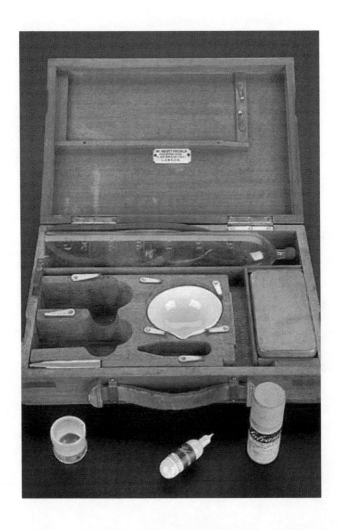

Salvarsan treatment kit for syphilis, Germany, 1909–1912.

he often replied: "For seven years of misfortune I had one moment of good luck".

Thanks to Salvarsan, syphilis, a nightmare that had lasted for more than 400 years, was no longer scary. Salvarsan (and later a better derivative neosalvarsan) wiped out half of the syphilis infections in Europe in 5 years. Salvarsan remained to be the magic bullet for syphilis for more than 30 years and was replaced by more effective and safer penicillin (the topic of Chapter 3) in the 1940s. Although no longer used nowadays, salvarsan was the first effective treatment for infectious diseases and indeed a miracle drug that changed the world.

2.6 Dr. Ehrlich's Philosophy – 4 G's

The salvarsan that Ehrlich developed marked the birth of chemotherapy. In addition to being the founder of pharmacology, Ehrlich has also been called the father of immunology. He received the Nobel Prize in Physiology or Medicine in 1908 due to his groundbreaking work in immunology. Ehrlich has made many remarkable achievements in different disciplines and is considered a giant among giants.

In his early careers, being a Jewish, for several years Ehrlich was not paid for his work. For a period of time, he even set up a personal laboratory in order to continue his research. He was obsessed with his research, and it was his entire life. Stacks of academic literature occupied his office. Books and magazines were placed everywhere. When he needed to explain one of his many theories and concepts, he would draw a diagram on items near him, including doors, the floor

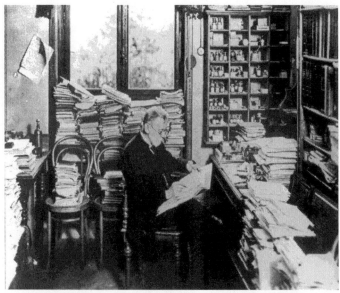

Paul Ehrlich around 1900 in his Frankfurt office.

of his laboratory, and even tablecloths at home. Fortunately, the family always had a supply of new tablecloths, thanks to his father-in-law who owned a textile factory.

Ehrlich summarized his philosophy of scientific discoveries as 4 G's:

Geld (money)

Geduld (patience)

Geschick (ingenuity)

Gluck (luck)

As Donald Kirsch commented on Ehrlich's 4G's in his book *The Drug Hunters*, "His formula was extremely prescient, since money, patience, ingenuity, and a heaping dose of serendipity remain essential ingredients for drug discovery to this very day."

CHAPTER 3

Penicillin – From Mysterious Mold to Miracle Drug

3.1 The Scottish Bacteriologist and his Mysterious Mold

It was a legendary story, which has been considered one of the most fascinating episodes in the history of medicine. The main character of the story was Alexander Fleming, a 47-year-old Scottish bacteriologist who had lived an unremarkable life by 1928. In the summer of 1928, Fleming and his family went to their country home for a month-long vacation. Before he left, due to his untidy habit, he did not clean a pile of petri dishes containing a bacterium (*Staphylococcus aureus*) that he had cultured.

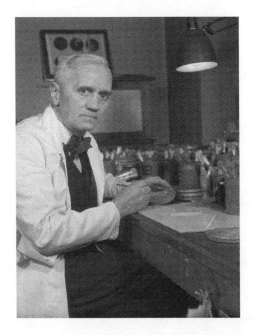

Alexander Fleming (1881-1955)

When he returned from his vacation, he came to his laboratory. It was Monday, September 3rd, 1928, a memorable day not only for Fleming but also for the history of medicine. He noticed that, while the bacteria in most dishes looked normal, one dish was contaminated with mold. Mold contamination would not have been something odd considering that microorganisms were everywhere, some of which could have settled on that dish. What was indeed unusual was that, in that dish, within the sea of *Staphylococcus aureus* (a type of Gram-positive bacteria that can cause disease) there was none of them surrounding the greenish mold, forming an empty ring. This suggested that the mold produced a substance that destroyed the bacteria around. After consulting with his colleagues, he learned that the mold was *Penicillium notatum*. Because of Fleming's experience and acute perception, instead of throwing away the ruined peri dish, he cultured that mold and named the substance "*penicillin*".

Penicillium notatum was a strange and rare mold. So how did this uncommon mold come to Fleming's dish? Among various rumors about this, the most convincing one was that it came from a laboratory downstairs and had been inadvertently blown into Fleming's *Staphylococcus aureus* culture dish. This was possible since a biologist was studying the connection between mold and asthma in the laboratory below

Fleming's, and one of the molds he studied was *Penicillium notatum*.

Two months later, Fleming tried to reproduce the original finding so that he could take a photograph to prove the original observation. It turned out to be a difficult task. When he put the mold directly on the colonies of *Staphylococcus aureus* and kept the dish at room temperature, there was no zone of inhibition and nothing noteworthy to photograph. With additional investigation, he found out that it worked only if he grew the mold first at room temperature, then seeded *Staphylococcus aureus* into the dish and put the Petri dish in the incubator. The underlying reason for this phenomenon is that the mold grows best at room temperature while the bacteria need body temperature to multiply. In addition, the mold *Penicillium notatum* only acts on bacteria that are young and actively multiplying. Apparently, there are several prerequisites before the occurrence of bacterial inhibition.

The temperature in the summer month usually is in favor of bacteria growth, which means that bacteria would age faster than the mold. Accordingly, the chance of seeing bacterial inhibition would be low since it only kills actively multiplying young bacteria.

So, for that particular dish with greenish mold and empty ring, the one Fleming saw on September 3rd, 1928, what happened and how could it happen?

It turned out that unreasonably low temperatures affected the weather in London for the first 9 days of August 1928, which gave the mold *Penicillium notatum* enough time to grow and meanwhile slowed down the growth of the bacteria *Staphylococcus aureus*. Then a heat wave hit on August 10. With increased temperature, the bacteria started to multiply, but the young bacteria were now facing the developed mold capable of killing them.

Penicillin, one of the most important medicines in the 20th century, was discovered after an incredible chain of serendipitous events took place in succession. As Vladimir Marko commented in his book, "Had Alexander Fleming left for vacation a week earlier or a week later, or if he had observed the bacteria in any other year, the discovery would never have been made." The extraordinary stroke of good luck made the story of penicillin discovery look more like fiction than fact.

Next, Fleming conducted several experiments to test the bacteria killing effect of penicillin. To his delight, penicillin not only effectively destroyed

Staphylococcus aureus, but also killed Streptococcus and the bacteria that cause meningitis, gonorrhea, and diphtheria. He published his findings in 1929. However, his work did not catch the attention of the medical community. One reason was likely the limited writing skills of Fleming; his papers were often short and lacked important details. Further, at 5 feet 5 inches, Fleming, nicknamed "little Flem", was not an impassioned speaker. His speech was quiet, halting, and boring. His seminars and lectures on the topic, same as his papers, were neither persuasive nor compelling, leaving the audience unengaged and unimpressed. Consequently, his papers on penicillin just sat on the shelf in the library, collecting dust, for almost a decade.

In addition, Fleming was a bacteriologist with limited knowledge of chemistry. He did not have the expertise and capability to take the next giant step of extracting penicillin and purifying it, let alone making it a medicine. During that time, Fleming sent his Penicillium mold to anyone who requested it, with the hope that other researchers could isolate penicillin for clinical use. For almost 10 years, no one was successful. Professor Harold Raistrick, a biochemist and fungal expert, declared "the production of penicillin for therapeutic purposes...almost impossible".

The entire story would have ended here. Penicillin would be labelled as a laboratory oddity and Fleming would have remained an obscure bacteriologist had three extremely talented scientists at Oxford University not picked up the work. Their story, as amazing as Fleming's, is the subject of the next section.

3.2 Three Brilliant Scientists and A Miracle Drug

There were three main characters in this story, and they could not be more different in terms of their background and personality.

Howard Walter Florey (1898-1968), the team leader, was born in Australia and received education in England. With extensive expertise in physiology and pathology, he joined the University of Oxford in 1935 as the department head of Dunn School of Pathology. Florey had a reputation of hard work, long hours and exacting standards. He worked every day, including Sunday. He was an excellent leader with great vision. In a very short time, Florey recruited a multidisciplinary team composed of talented and enthusiastic researchers. Among his first hires was the biochemist Ernst Boris Chain, another key member of the penicillin project.

Ernst Boris Chain (1906-1979) was from Germany and a Russian-German-Jewish descent. With brushed back curly black hair and a black moustache, at first glance Chain looked like Albert Einstein. In 1933, shortly after he graduated in biochemistry from University in Berlin, Nazis came to power. The same year, Chain left his homeland for England, with £10 in his pocket. He joined Florey's team in 1937.

The third member was Norman George Heatley (1911- 2004), an English gentleman and a skilled chemist. He was the exact opposite of Chain in many aspects, although both were sharp and brilliant researchers. Chain was abrupt, abrasive and acutely sensitive, while Heatley was quiet and modest. Heatley wrote meticulous notes while Chain took few notes in his notebook. Heatley was reluctant to seek credit while Chain fought constantly for it. Despite their personality incompatibility, things were under control, thanks to their leader Florey, who was an absolute

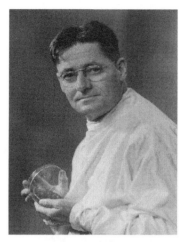

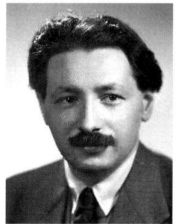

Howard Walter Florey (Upper) and Ernst Boris Chain (Lower). None of Norman Heatley's photos are in the public domain. So, I am not able to share it here due to copyright restrain.

wizard at running a large laboratory filled with talented but quirky scientists.

One research direction that Chain worked on, under Florey's guidance, was bacterial antagonism. Chain read about 200 references on this topic but did not find relevant information. One day in 1938, by sheer luck, Chain came across Fleming's paper on penicillin. The paper captured both Chain and Florey's interest, and they started penicillin research when a grant came in.

It turned out to be an extremely challenging project. First, isolating and purifying penicillin, an unstable substance, was not easy. With numerous trial and error, this challenging task was solved by Chain. The key components of the successful technique that Chain established lied in controlling the pH of the "juice," reducing the sample's temperature, and evaporating the product over and over (essentially freeze-drying it). Another daunting task was to produce enough penicillin. In Fleming's original mold sample, there were two units of penicillin per milliliter of solution. The average daily dose of penicillin is approximately 15,000,000 units. What does that mean? It means that if we use Fleming's petri dishes, we would need an astonishing quantity of dishes that together can cover several football fields in order to get a daily dose.

The task of efficiently producing penicillin fell on Heatley's shoulder. The mold *Penicillium notatum* needs oxygen, so a sufficient air supply is important. Heatley discovered that the mold would continue to grow and produce more penicillin if the culture medium was constantly replaced. The team tried culturing the mold *Penicillium notatum* in all kinds of cylindrical vessels, such as empty cake tins, gas cans, milk churns, bedpans, etc. Bedpan turned out to be the winner. The production of penicillin significantly improved.

In May 1940, Florey and his team carried out a vital experiment, in which 8 mice were infected with deadly streptococcus, one hour later four of them were given a solution of the dark brown powder containing penicillin while the other four received no treatment as the blank control.

Heatley recorded the experiment in his diary:

"After supper with some friends, I returned to the lab and met the professor to give a final dose of penicillin to two of the mice. The 'controls' were looking very sick, but the two treated mice seemed very well. I stayed at the lab until 3:45 a.m., by which time all four control animals were dead."

On returning home, Heatley realized that in haste and darkness, he had put his underpants on back to front, and noted this in his diary too.

The team, albeit all were thrilled with the astonishing results, reacted as differently as their personalities. Chain danced around the laboratory with excitement. Heatley attributed the success to the misarrangement of his underpants that occurred the day before. Florey, calm and reserved as usual, modestly said, "it looks quite promising". He also brought Chain and Heatley back to earth by saying, "man is 3000 times the size of the mouse".

After the successful animal experiments, Florey decided to administer penicillin to humans. This was not a trivial task as they needed sufficient quantity of penicillin. To address this need, Heatley designed a fermentation vessel of similar shape of Bedpan. Based on Heatley's drawings, one of Florey's friends, who owned a ceramic factory, manufactured several hundreds of bedpans for mold cultivation.

The Oxford laboratory literally was turned into a penicillin factory. A team of "penicillin girls" was employed, at £ 2 per week, to cultivate and look after the fermentation. Finally, the team had enough penicillin and was ready to test its antibacterial effect in humans.

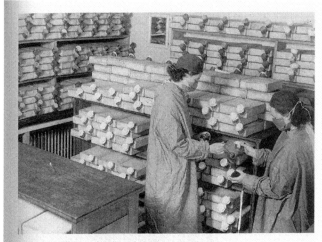

"Penicillin Girls" tending the Heatley-designed vessels for growing penicillin mould at the Sir William Dunn School in Oxford. COURTESY OF NORMAN HEATLEY

"Penicillin girls" were growing penicillin mold at the Sir William Dunn School in Oxford.

The first patient was Albert Alexander, a 43-year-old Oxford policeman, who was near death's door from a severe infection which resulted from a scratch while pruning a rose bush. There were huge abscesses affecting his eyes, face, and lungs. After the first few doses of penicillin, he made a remarkable recovery within days. Unfortunately, the supply of penicillin ran out several days later. As a large percentage of penicillin was excreted in the urine in its original state, efforts had been made to collect every drop of urine from the patient, send it to the pathology department, extract penicillin from the urine, and then send back to the clinic. Unfortunately, this was still not enough. A month later, Alexander relapsed and died. Later, several other similar hopeless cases were treated with penicillin, and all patients recovered.

The powerful antibacterial effect of penicillin was indisputable. The rate limiting step was penicillin production, which could not be addressed by the modestly equipped pathology department. Florey approached several British companies, but none could help because there was a war going on and the chemical industry was fully absorbed for more urgent priorities. Recognizing that large-scale production of penicillin was out of question in Britain, Florey decided to try his luck in the United States. The journey of penicillin in the United States, another interesting story, is the topic of the next section.

3.3 Unprecedented Multi-party Collaboration

Florey and Heatley traveled to the United States in the summer of 1941 to seek help. It was war time. There were no direct or safe connections between London and New York. They took a dangerous flight in a blacked-out Pan-Am Clipper seaplane. It took them one week to reach their destiny; during the trip Florey and Heatley were constantly worried that temperature change would ruin their precious *Penicillium* mold and the penicillin samples in their briefcase. Also worried that the Nazis would take the mold if they were caught, Florey and Heatley rubbed the mold into their coats. Fortunately, the mold survived the trip.

After they arrived in the United States, through Florey's connections, they were introduced to the Northern Regional Research Laboratory (NRRL) in Peoria, Illinois, where significant improvement in penicillin production process took place. Researchers in NRRL recognized that growing the mold in submerged culture, instead of the surface of a nutrient medium, was a superior method. However, the *Penicillum* stain that Florey brought did not respond well to the submerged culture. To find a better yielding strain of mold, a global search was underway, and several thousand mold specimens from various places were sent to NRRL. Interestingly, the mold strain that stood out among all was not from the soils of a distant locale, but rather from a rotten cantaloupe found at a local Peoria market. Mary Hunt, the lady who brought the cantaloupe specimen, earned the nickname "Moldy Mary".

In addition, NRRL researchers significantly boosted penicillin yield by modifying the method, including the addition of corn-steep liquor, an abundant by-product of the corn wet milling process, to the fermentation medium. The price of corn steep liquor was once inflated because of its use in mold cultivation.

While Heatley stayed in Peoria and worked with NRRL staff on optimization of penicillin production process, Florey visited various pharmaceutical companies to try to raise their interest. To his disappointment, the immediate responses from the companies were not promising. Florey next visited his old friend Alfred Richards, who was the chair of the Committee on Medical Research of the Office of Scientific Research and Development. Bearing the trust of Florey's judgment about the potential value of penicillin, Richards called a meeting among the representatives of National research Council, the U.S. Department of Agriculture, and several companies. While the first meeting was not productive, the second conference was definitely more decisive because it was held in December 1941, ten days after the Pearl Harbor attack and the U.S. entry into World War II. Merck, Squibb, Abbott, and Pfizer were the first to participate in the penicillin project. Later, many other companies joined.

Even though the updated method optimized by NRRL improved penicillin yield, scaling it up to a manufacturing scale was not easy. As John Smith from Pfizer commented, "The mold as temperamental as an opera singer, the yields are low, the isolation is difficult, the extraction is murder, the purification invites disaster, and the assay is unsatisfactory." Despite numerous obstacles, pharmaceutical and chemical companies played a crucial role in solving all problems inherent in the scale-up process.

To supply the Allied troops with enough penicillin, the American War Production Board (WPB) granted top priority to all participating companies on materials and other suppliers to speed up penicillin mass production. One goal was to provide an adequate supply of penicillin for the proposed D-day invasion of Europe. Wartime patriotism stimulated the work on penicillin. Albert Elder wrote to manufacturers in 1943: "You are urged to impress upon every worker in your plant that penicillin produced today will be saving the life of someone in a few days or curing the disease of someone now incapacitated. Put up slogans in your plant! Place notice in pay envelopes! Create an enthusiasm for the job down to the lowest worker in your plant."

By the end of 1943, penicillin production was the second highest priority at the War Department, preceded only by atomic bomb development. By that year, allied troops received sufficient penicillin. Penicillin not only safely and effectively treated syphilis (a disease described in Chapter 2), but also

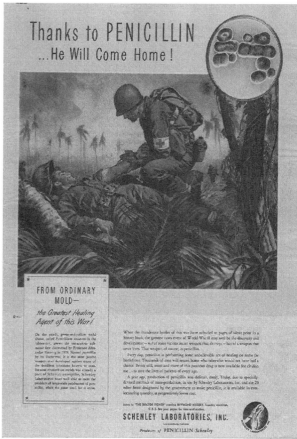

A 1944 WW2 poster featuring a wounded US soldier being administered pencillin by a male military nurse in the jungle. An inset of cells on a culture plate is to the top right hand corner of the image. Advertisement by Schenley Laboratories Medic Helping Soldier Art.

demonstrated remarkable antibacterial effect against various other infections. A miracle drug indeed. Countless lives were saved during WWII.

In the beginning, because of the limited supply of penicillin, priority was given to military use. The news of this miracle drug began to reach the public. Chester Keefer, the government official who oversaw the distribution of penicillin, was besieged with pleas for penicillin. A newspaper in Oct 1943 stated: "Many laymen -husbands, wives, parents, brothers, sisters, friends – beg Dr. Keefer for penicillin. In every case the petitioner is told to arrange that a full dossier on the patient's condition be sent by the doctor in charge. When this is received, the decision is made on a medical, not an emotional basis."

Fortunately, with unprecedented multi-party collaboration and commitment, penicillin mass production became a reality. Production of penicillin in the United States reached 21 billion units in 1943, and the number jumped to 1,663 billion units in 1944, then leaped to more than 6.8 trillion units in 1945. In March 1945, the American government was able to remove all restrictions, and penicillin was available to civilians. As Florey said in 1949, "too high a tribute cannot be paid to the enterprise and energy with which the American manufacturing firms tackled the large-scale production of the drug. Had it not been for their efforts there would certainly not have been sufficient penicillin by D-Day in Normandy in 1944 to treat all severe casualties, both British and American."

3.4 Unsung Heroes

It's clear that turning penicillin into a miracle drug was a joint effort, with both Fleming and the Oxford team being indispensable. However, it was Fleming who became the spokesperson in front of the media and got most of the glory, while the Oxford team was shunned the public attention. The Fleming myth, as it has been called, was promoted by the publicity machine at St. Mary's Hospital, where Fleming worked. Fleming never clarified some of the grossly exaggerated claims made by St. Mary's in the press.

Florey kept silent in terms of the credit for the penicillin discovery, which made Chain really upset as he felt that Fleming had stolen the spotlight and all the credit. Another thing that deteriorated the relationship between Chain and Florey was the patent of penicillin. Chain had an industrial background and urged Florey to patent penicillin. However, Florey, as a physician abiding by Hipporates' oath, was hesitant to make profit from a medical discovery. Their American partners had no such concern and quickly patented the production process of penicillin. The reality of Britain paying Americans for their own discovery of penicillin was a brutal one for Chain to swallow. It became more and more difficult for these two intellectual giants to work together. Chain left Oxford in 1949, and he did not return to the Dunn school for 30 years.

The lack of recognition of the Oxford team was partially corrected in 1945, when Fleming, Florey, and Chain were awarded the Nobel Prize in Physiology or Medicine for their work on penicillin. Heatley did not get credit for his contribution for more than 4 decades till 1990, when he was awarded an Honorary Doctorate of Medicine from Oxford University; this was an unusual distinction as it was the first given to a non-medic in Oxford's 800-year history.

Based on rough estimation, the development of penicillin saved over 80 million lives. The discovery of penicillin marks a true turning point in human history. Many school kids can recite the basics of the story of Fleming and penicillin; but probably none of them has heard of the Oxford team (Florey, Chain, and Heatley), the undervalued heroes.   Ultimately, the story of penicillin is a saga involving people from various backgrounds during a critical time of need - from ordinary citizens and technicians to dedicated researchers and industry partners. The combined effort may be the most important message to remember, then and now.

BIBLIOGRAPHY

This book was written based on information from various sources, including drug history books, review articles, websites, blogs, magazine interviews, etc. Here I only list several key references.

Key References

- Bosch, Fèlix; Rosich, Laia. The Contributions of Paul Ehrlich to Pharmacology: A Tribute on the Occasion of the Centenary of His Nobel Prize. Pharmacology 2008;82:171–179.
- Frith, John. Syphilis - Its Early History and Treatment Until Penicillin, and the Debate on its Origins. Journal of Military and Veterans' Health 2012; 20(4): 49-58.
- Hager, Thomas. *Ten Drugs.* Abrams Press, New York, 2019
- Lee, MR. Plants Against Malaria Part 1: Cinchona or the Peruvian Bark. J R Coll Physicians Edinb 2002; 32:189–196.
- Li, Jie J. *Laughing Gas, Viagra, and Lipitor.* Oxford University Press, Inc: New York, 2006.
- Marko, Vladimir. *From Aspirin to Viagra.* Springer Nature Switzerland, 2020
- Kirsch, Donald R, Ogas, Ogi. *The Drug Hunters.* Arcade Publishing, New York, 2018
- Rocco, Fiammetta. *The Miraculous Fever Tree.* Harper Collins, 2003.
- Sherman, Irwin W. *Drugs That Changed the World.* CRC Press: Boca Raton, FL, 2017.
- Sherman, Irwin W. *Twelve Diseases That Changed Our World.* ASM Press: Washington, DC, 2007.

Word Puzzle

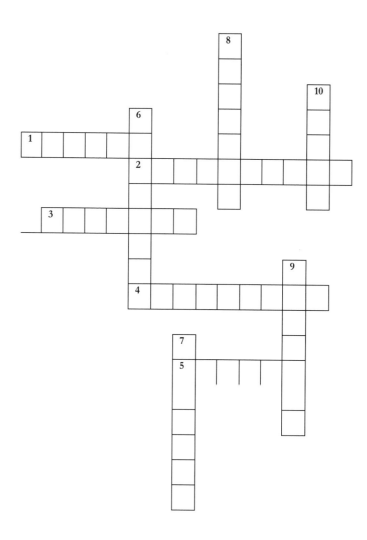

Clues

Across:

1. Oxford team lead (last name only) who played a key role in turning a substance from mold into a miracle drug.
2. A substance produced by the mold *Penicillinum motatum* which can kill many types of bacteria.
3. A wonder drug that is extracted from the bark of the cinchona tree.
4. Dr. Ehrlich's magic bullet.
5. An unlucky adventurer (last name only) who provided the best quality cinchona seeds to the Dutch.

Down:

6. A scary disease which was believed to be brought to the old world by Columbus and his sailors. The first outbreak was in 1495.
7. A Scottish bacteriologist (last name only) who discovered a miracle drug after an incredible chain of accidental events took place.
8. A scientific genius (last name only) who used his magic bullet to successfully cure one of the most feared diseases in Europe for several centuries.
9. A terrible disease transmitted by mosquitoes.
10. One of the Oxford team members who was a Jewish refugee.

CHEMICAL STRUCTURE

Quinine

Salvarsan (Ehrlich's 606)

Penicillin G

ADDITIONAL NOTE

Thank you again for reading this book. I hope you like these short stories and find the information useful. Book #2, *"The Unforgettables"* will be released at Amazon in December 2024.

Made in the USA
Middletown, DE
03 September 2024

60099850R00061